THE COMPLETE MEDITERRANEAN DIET WEIGHT LOSS SOLUTION 2024

Delicious Quick and Easy Recipes to Lower High Blood Pressure, Lose Your Weight Naturally and Improve Your Overall Health

Dr. Raphael Rachelle

TABLE OF CONTENTS

ENCOURAGEMENT

Positive Mindset: Approach this journey with positivity, celebrating small victories along the way. Focus on adopting a lifestyle that nurtures both physical and mental well-being.

Diverse and Delicious: Savor the richness of the Mediterranean Diet's diverse flavors. Enjoy the journey of exploring fresh, whole foods, and let the deliciousness of each meal be a source of joy.

Mindful Eating: Practice mindful eating by paying attention to your body 's suggestions.. Recognize when you're hungry and when you're satisfied, allowing for a more intuitive and sustainable approach to weight management.

Hydration Matters: Remember the importance of staying hydrated. Water is a key component in promoting overall health and aiding in weight loss. Consider adding flavor with teas made from herbs and infused water.

Joyful Movement: Find physical activities that bring you joy. Whether it's walking, dancing, or practicing yoga, choose exercises that align with your interests. Consistent movement contributes not only to weight loss but also to improved mood and energy levels.

Support System: Build a supportive network around you. Share your goals, challenges, and successes with friends, family, or online communities Having a support system can make the journey more joyful and long-lasting..

Patience and Consistency: Remember that losing weight is a slow process.. Keep in mind that losing weight is a gradual process. Be gentle with yourself and constant in your efforts. Sustainable changes take time, but they lead to lasting results.

Celebrate Achievements: Celebrate not only the number on the scale but also non-scale victories. Acknowledge improvements in energy levels, mood, and overall well-being. These achievements are equally significant on your journey to a healthier you.

INTRODUCTION

In the bustling heart of a modern city, where the fast-paced rhythm often dictated lifestyle choices, Emily found herself at a crossroads. Tired of the constant cycle of fad diets and fleeting health resolutions, she yearned for a sustainable and holistic approach to weight loss. It was then that she stumbled upon "The Complete Mediterranean Diet Weight Loss Solution."

As Emily delved into the pages of this transformative guide, she discovered not just a collection of recipes but a roadmap to a vibrant and nourishing lifestyle. The book became her compass, guiding her through the colorful and flavorful world of Mediterranean cuisine. The emphasis on fresh, whole foods, the joy of mindful eating, and the celebration of life's simple pleasures resonated with her on a profound level.

Armed with newfound knowledge, Emily embarked on a culinary adventure, creating delectable meals that not only satisfied her taste buds but fueled her journey to a healthier self. The Mediterranean Diet became her ally, transforming her relationship with food and exercise. It wasn't just about shedding pounds; it was about embracing a lifestyle that promoted well-being, inside and out.

As weeks turned into months, Emily's story unfolded as a testament to the power of the Mediterranean Diet.

Her increased energy levels, improved mood, and the gradual but sustainable weight loss were not just markers of success; they were the tangible results of a commitment to a balanced and joyful way of living.

This is the story of how "The Complete Mediterranean Diet Weight Loss Solution" became more than a book for Emily—it became the catalyst for her success, empowering her to reclaim control over her health and rewrite the narrative of her life.

Overview of the Mediterranean diet

1. **Emphasis on Fresh, Whole Foods:**

   - The Mediterranean diet focuses on consuming a variety of fresh, whole foods, including fruits, vegetables, nuts, seeds, legumes, and whole grains.

2. **Healthy Fats:**

   - Rather than avoiding fats, the diet promotes healthy fats, especially those found in olive oil, nuts, and fatty fish. These fats are rich in monounsaturated and omega-3 fatty acids.

3. **Lean Proteins:**

   - Protein sources include lean meats, poultry, fish, and plant-based options like legumes and tofu.

4. **Moderate Dairy:**

   - Dairy products, particularly in the form of cheese and yogurt, are consumed in moderation.

5. **Limited Red Meat:**

   - Red meat is limited in the Mediterranean diet, with a preference for leaner protein sources.

6. **Herbs and Spices:**

   - Herbs and spices are freely utilized to flavor foods, decreasing the need for salt.

7. **Wine in Moderation:**

   - While not mandatory, moderate consumption of red wine, especially during meals, is a characteristic feature in some Mediterranean cultures.

8. **Focus on Plant-Based:**

   - The diet places a strong emphasis on plant-based foods, contributing to high fiber intake and a variety of essential nutrients.

9. **Regular Physical Activity:**

   - In addition to dietary choices, the Mediterranean lifestyle includes regular physical activity, such as walking and other forms of exercise.

10.   **Social and Family Aspect:**

- Meals are often seen as a social activity, with an emphasis on enjoying food in the company of others.

11.   **Health Benefits:**

- Numerous studies have linked the Mediterranean diet to various health benefits, including reduced risk of heart disease, improved weight management, and potential positive effects on cognitive function.

Importance of Weight Loss for Overall Health

1. Ovary syndrome (PCOS) in women. **Cardiovascular Health:**

   - Excess body weight, particularly abdominal fat, is linked to an increased risk of cardiovascular diseases such as heart attack and stroke. Weight loss can improve blood pressure, cholesterol levels, and overall cardiovascular function.

2. **Type 2 Diabetes Prevention and Management:**

   - Maintaining a healthy weight is crucial for preventing the onset of type 2 diabetes. For those already diagnosed, weight loss can help manage blood sugar levels and reduce the need for medication.

3. **Joint Health:**

   - Carrying excess weight places additional stress on joints, particularly in the knees, hips, and lower back. Weight loss can alleviate this stress, reducing the risk of joint pain and arthritis.

4. **Improved Respiratory Function:**

   - Obesity is associated with respiratory issues such as sleep apnea and decreased lung function. Weight loss can lead to improved respiratory health and reduce the severity of breathing disorders.

5. **Cancer Risk Reduction:**

   - Some types of cancer, including breast, colon, and prostate cancer, are more prevalent in individuals with obesity. Weight loss may lower the risk and improve outcomes for those undergoing cancer treatments.

6. **Enhanced Mental Health:**

   - Achieving and maintaining a healthy weight has been shown to im prove mental health. It can boost self-esteem, reduce symptoms of depression and anxiety, and contribute to an overall sense of well-being.

7. **Liver Health:**

   - Obesity is linked to non-alcoholic fatty liver disease (NAFLD).. Weight loss can help improve liver function and prevent the progression of liver disease.

Hormonal Balance:

- Obesity can disrupt hormonal balance, leading to conditions such as polycystic ovary syndrome (PCOS) in women and reduced testosterone levels in men. Weight loss can help restore hormonal equilibrium.

8. **Quality of Sleep:**

- Obesity is a risk factor for sleep disorders such as sleep apnea. Losing weight can improve sleep quality and reduce the severity of sleep-related breathing problems.

9. **Longevity and Overall Life Quality:**

- Maintaining a healthy weight is linked to increased life expectancy. Additionally, weight loss can enhance the quality of life by improving mobility, energy levels, and overall vitality.

Core Principles of the Mediterranean Diet

1. **Emphasis on Plant-Based Foods:**

   - The majority of the diet consists of plant-based foods, including fruits, vegetables, legumes, nuts, and seeds. These foods provide a rich source of vitamins, minerals, fiber, and antioxidants.

2. **Olive Oil as the Primary Fat:**

   - In the Mediterranean diet, olive oil is the predominant source of dietary fat. It contains monounsaturated fats, which have been linked to heart health. Olive oil is used for cooking, dressing salads, and flavoring various dishes.

3. **Moderate Consumption of Fish and Poultry:**

   - In the Mediterranean diet, fish and poultry are chosen over red meat. Fatty fish, such as salmon and mackerel, are particularly emphasized due to their omega-3 fatty acid content.

4. **Limited Red Meat Intake:**

   - Red meat, including beef and lamb, is consumed in moderation. The diet encourages lean protein sources and limits the intake of processed meats.

5. **Dairy in Moderation:**

   - Moderate amounts of dairy products, such as cheese and yogurt, ar e included.. These provide calcium and probiotics while avoiding excessive saturated fat intake.

6. **Abundance of Whole Grains:**

   - Whole grains, such as whole wheat, barlcy, oats, and brown rice, are staples in the Mediterranean diet. They are rich in fiber, vitamins, and minerals.

7. **Fresh Fruits and Vegetables Daily:**

   - A wide variety of fresh fruits and vegetables are consumed daily, providing essential nutrients, antioxidants, and fiber. These foods are a central focus of every meal.

8. **Nuts and Seeds as Snacks:**

   - Nuts and seeds, such as almonds, walnuts, and sunflower seeds, are included as healthy snacks. They contribute healthy fats, protein, and micronutrients.

9. Herbs and Spices for Flavor:

- Herbs and spices are freely utilized to flavor dishes, which reduces the need for excessive salt..Popular spices and herbs include basil, oregano, rosemary, and garlic.

10. Moderate Consumption of Wine:

- While not mandatory, moderate consumption of red wine is a characteristic feature of the Mediterranean diet, particularly during meals. This is believed to have cardiovascular benefits.

11. Social Eating and Enjoyment of Meals:

- Meals are seen as a social activity in Mediterranean cultures. Taking time to enjoy and savor meals with family and friends is an integral part of the lifestyle.

12. Regular Physical Activity:

- The Mediterranean lifestyle includes regular physical activity, such as walking, cycling, and other forms of exercise. Physical activity complements the diet in promoting overall health.

Benefits beyond Weight Loss

1. **Heart Health:**

   - The Mediterranean diet is renowned for its positive impact on cardiovascular health. The emphasis on olive oil, fish, nuts, and whole grains contributes to lower cholesterol levels, reduced blood pressure, and a decreased risk of heart disease.

2. **Reduced Risk of Type 2 Diabetes:**

   - The diet's focus on whole, unprocessed foods, and the inclusion of complex carbohydrates helps regulate blood sugar levels, reducing the risk of type 2 diabetes.

3. **Improved Cognitive Function:**

   - Studies suggest that the Mediterranean diet, rich in antioxidants and omega-3 fatty acids, may support brain health and reduce the risk of cognitive decline and neurodegenerative diseases.

4. **Inflammation Reduction:**

   - The diet's abundance of anti-inflammatory foods, such as fruits, vegetables, and fatty fish, may help reduce chronic inflammation, a factor associated with various diseases, including arthritis and certain cancers.

5. **Cancer Prevention:**

   - Some components of the Mediterranean diet, such as a high intake of fruits, vegetables, and olive oil, are associated with a lower risk of certain cancers, including breast and colorectal cancers.

6. **Improved Weight Management:**

   - While weight loss is one aspect, the Mediterranean diet supports healthy weight management over the long term. The emphasis on nutrient-dense, satisfying foods helps control appetite and prevents overeating.

7. **Better Digestive Health:**

   - The diet's high fiber content, derived from fruits, vegetables, and whole grains, promotes a healthy digestive system and may reduce the risk of conditions such as constipation and diverticulitis.

8. **Enhanced Mood and Mental Health:**

   - The consumption of omega-3 fatty acids found in fish, as well as nutrient-rich foods, may positively influence mood and mental well-being, potentially reducing the risk of depression and anxiety.

9. **Longevity:**

- Studies have suggested that adherence to the Mediterranean diet is associated with increased life expectancy, likely due to its protective effects against chronic diseases.

10. **Improved Sleep Quality:**

- Some components of the diet, such as magnesium-rich foods and the promotion of overall health, may contribute to better sleep quality and patterns.

11. **Better Skin Health:**

- The inclusion of foods rich in antioxidants and healthy fats, such as olive oil and fatty fish, may contribute to improved skin health, reducing the signs of aging and promoting a youthful complexion.

12. **Balanced Hormones:**

- The diet's emphasis on nutrient-dense foods, healthy fats, and a balanced intake of carbohydrates may contribute to hormonal balance, especially in conditions like polycystic

Nutritional Components of the Diet

1. **Healthy Fats:**

   - **Olive Oil:** A primary source of fat in the Mediterranean diet, rich in monounsaturated fats and antioxidants.

   - **Nuts and Seeds:** Provide healthy fats, including omega-3 fatty acids (found in walnuts and flaxseeds) and various beneficial nutrients.

   - **Fatty Fish:** Such as salmon, mackerel, and sardines, which are high in omega-3 fatty acids.

2. **Lean Proteins:**

   - **Fish and Seafood:** Protein and omega-3 fatty acids are abundant in fish and seafood..

   - **Poultry:** Especially chicken and turkey, providing a lean source of protein.

   - **Legumes:** Beans, lentils, and chickpeas are all good plant-based protein sources.

3. **Whole Grains:**

- **Whole Wheat:** Including whole wheat bread and pasta.

- **Brown Rice:** A staple in the diet, providing fiber and essential nutrients.

- **Quinoa, Barley, and Oats:** Additional whole grains that add variety and nutritional value.

4. **Abundance of Fruits and Vegetables:**

- A wide variety of colorful fruits and vegetables provide essential vitamins, minerals, fiber, and antioxidants.

5. **Dairy in Moderation:**

- **Greek Yogurt:** A common dairy product in moderation, rich in protein and probiotics.

- **Cheese:** Consumed in moderation, providing calcium and additional nutrients.

6. **Herbs and Spices:**

- **Basil, Rosemary, Oregano, and Garlic:** Used liberally to flavor dishes, reducing the need for excessive salt.

7. **Wine in Moderation:**

- **Red Wine:** Consumed in moderation, offering antioxidants and potential cardiovascular benefits.

8. **Fruits and Nuts as Snacks:**

- **Fresh Fruits:** A common and nutritious snack.

- **Nuts and Seeds:** Such as almonds and sunflower seeds, providing healthy fats and additional nutrients.

9. **Water and Herbal Teas:**

- Hydration is often maintained through water and herbal teas, contributing to overall health.

10. **Moderate Sweets and Desserts:**

- **Honey and Fresh Fruit:** Used as natural sweeteners.

- **Pastries and Sweets:** Consumed in moderation.

11. **Regular Physical Activity:**

- While not a dietary component, physical activity is a crucial part of the Mediterranean lifestyle, contributing to overall health.

How the Mediterranean diet Supports Weight Loss

1. **Rich in Whole, Nutrient-Dense Foods:**

   - The diet emphasizes whole, minimally processed foods such as fruits, vegetables, whole grains, lean proteins, and healthy fats. These foods are nutrient-dense, providing essential vitamins, minerals, and fiber, which promote satiety and reduce overall calorie intake.

2. **Healthy Fats for Satiety:**

   - The inclusion of olive oil, nuts, and fatty fish provides healthy monounsaturated fats and omega-3 fatty acids. These fats enhance the feeling of fullness and satisfaction, reducing the likelihood of overeating.

3. **Balanced Macronutrient Profile:**

   - The Mediterranean diet maintains a balanced distribution of macronutrients, including a moderate intake of carbohydrates, proteins, and fats. This balance helps regulate blood sugar levels, preventing energy crashes that can lead to cravings and overeating.

4. **High Fiber Content:**

- The abundance of fruits, vegetables, and whole grains in the diet contributes to a high fiber intake. Fiber promotes digestive health, regulates appetite, and helps control blood sugar levels, all of which are beneficial for weight management.

5. **Lean Protein Sources:**

- The diet includes lean protein sources such as fish, poultry, legumes, and plant-based proteins. Protein is known for its role in promoting fullness and preserving lean muscle mass, especially important during weight loss.

6. **Reduced Red Meat Consumption:**

- Red meat is limited in the Mediterranean diet, and when consumed, it is often lean and in moderation. This restriction can help reduce overall calorie intake and saturated fat consumption.

7. **Social and Mindful Eating:**

- The Mediterranean lifestyle places importance on social and mindful eating. Enjoying meals with family and friends, savoring flavors, and being present during meals can contribute to a more conscious approach to eating, reducing the likelihood of overeating.

8. **Regular Physical Activity:**

- While not a direct dietary component, the Mediterranean lifestyle encourages regular physical activity. Incorporating exercise into daily routines contributes to overall calorie expenditure and enhances weight loss efforts.

9. **Reduced Processed Foods and Sugars:**

- The diet minimizes the intake of processed foods, refined sugars, and sugary beverages. This helps regulate blood sugar levels, reduces calorie-dense but nutrient-poor foods, and supports weight loss.

10. **Long-Term Sustainability:**

- The Mediterranean diet is not a short-term or restrictive plan, making it more sustainable for long-term weight management. It encourages a balanced and enjoyable approach to eating, reducing the likelihood of yo-yo dieting.

11. **Potential Metabolic Benefits:**

- Some studies suggest that the Mediterranean diet may have positive effects on metabolic health, including improved insulin sensitivity, which can be beneficial for weight management.

Creating a Mediterranean Pantry

1. Oils and Fats:

- Extra Virgin Olive Oil

- Canola Oil (for cooking)

- Nuts (e.g., almonds, walnuts)

- Seeds (e.g., sunflower seeds, flaxseeds)

2. Whole Grains:

- Whole Wheat Pasta

- Brown Rice

- Quinoa

- Bulgur

- Farro

- Whole Grain Couscous

3. Legumes:

- Lentils

- Chickpeas

- Cannellini Beans

- Black Beans

4. Canned and Jarred Goods:

- Canned Tomatoes (diced, crushed, and whole)

- Tomato Paste
- Artichoke Hearts (in water, canned or jarred)
- Olives (various types, such as Kalamata and green)
- Roasted Red Peppers

5. Dried Herbs and Spices:

- Dried Oregano
- Dried Basil
- Dried Thyme
- Rosemary
- Cumin
- Coriander
- Paprika
- Red Pepper Flakes
- Ground Cinnamon

6. Fresh Herbs:

- Basil
- Parsley
- Mint
- Rosemary
- Thyme

- Dill

7. Grains and Flours:

- Whole Wheat Flour
- Almond Flour
- Polenta (cornmeal)
- Bread Crumbs (whole grain)
- Rolled Oats

8. Nuts and Seeds:

- Almonds
- Walnuts
- Pine Nuts
- Chia Seeds
- Flaxseeds
- Sesame Seeds

9. Canned Fish and Seafood:

- Canned Tuna (in water)
- Canned Salmon
- Anchovies

10. Dairy and Dairy Alternatives:

- Greek Yogurt

- Feta Cheese
- Parmesan Cheese
- Goat Cheese
- Almond Milk

11. Proteins:

- Skinless Chicken Breast
- Lean Turkey
- Eggs

12. Fresh Produce:

- Tomatoes
- Bell Peppers
- Cucumbers
- Spinach
- Kale
- Zucchini
- Eggplant
- Onions
- Garlic
- Lemons
- Oranges

13. Beverages:

- Red Wine (optional, for moderate consumption)
- Herbal Teas

14. Sweeteners:

- Honey
- Maple Syrup

15. Miscellaneous:

- Capers
- Vinegar (red wine vinegar, balsamic vinegar)
- Dijon Mustard
- Whole Olives

Tips:

- Choose whole and minimally processed foods.
- Opt for extra virgin olive oil as your primary cooking oil.
- Purchase canned goods with no added salt or low sodium content.
- Consider buying in bulk to save money.
- Regularly check your pantry to restock perishables and ensure freshness.

Food to Include, Limit and Avoid

Foods to Include:

1. **Fruits and Vegetables:**

   - Include a range of brightly colored fruits and vegetables in your re gular diet.. These are rich in vitamins, minerals, and antioxidants.

2. **Whole Grains:**

   - Choose whole grains such as quinoa, brown rice, whole wheat, and oats for fiber and sustained energy.

3. **Healthy Fats:** Incorporate sources of healthy fats like olive oil, nuts, seeds, and avocados these fats help with heart health and satiety.

4. **Lean Proteins:**

   - Opt for lean protein sources, including fish, poultry, legumes, and tofu. Fish, particularly fatty fish such as salmon, is high in omega-3 fatty acids.

5. **Dairy or Dairy Alternatives:**

   - Include moderate amounts of dairy or dairy alternatives like Greek yogurt and cheese for calcium and probiotics.

6. **Herbs and Spices:**

   - Flavor your dishes with herbs and spices like basil, oregano, thyme, and garlic, reducing the need for excessive salt.

7. **Water:**

   - Stay hydrated with water. Water is the primary beverage in the Mediterranean Diet.

8. **Moderate Red Wine (Optional):**

   - If you consume alcohol, enjoy red wine in moderation. It's a common component of the Mediterranean lifestyle.

Foods to Limit:

1. **Red Meat:**

   - Limit your intake of red and processed meats. Choose leaner cuts and smaller serving sizes.

2. **Processed Foods:**

   - Reduce the intake of processed and packaged foods, as they often contain added sugars, unhealthy fats, and preservatives.

3. **Refined Grains:**

   - Limit the consumption of refined grains such as white bread and white rice. Choose whole grains for better nutritional value.

4. **Added Sugars:**

   - Keep an eye out for extra sugars in your diet..

5. **Saturated Fats:**

   - Limit saturated fats found in butter and full-fat dairy. Choose healthy fats such as olive oil.

Foods to Avoid:

1. **Trans Fats:**

   - Trans fats present in partially hydrogenated oils should be avoided. Check food labels, and steer clear of products containing Trans fats.

2. **Highly Processed Foods:**

   - Avoid highly processed and refined foods, as they often lack essential nutrients and can contribute to weight gain.

3. **Excessive Salt:**

   - Limit excessive salt intake. Instead of salt, use herbs and spices to flavor your dish.

4. **Sugary Beverages:**

   - Sugary drinks, such as sodas and fruit juices, should be avoided. Instead, drink water, herbal teas, or infused water.

5. **Fried Foods:**

   - Minimize the consumption of fried foods. Cooking methods that are healthier to use include grilling, baking, and sautéing.

Nourishing Breakfast Recipes

Mediterranean Avocado Toast

Ingredients:

- Whole grain bread
- Ripe avocado
- Cherry tomatoes, sliced
- Extra virgin olive oil
- Fresh basil, chopped
- Salt and pepper to taste

Instructions:

1. Toast the whole grain bread slices.
2. Spread the mashed avocado equally on the toasted bread.
3. Arrange sliced cherry tomatoes on top.
4. Drizzle with extra virgin olive oil.
5. Sprinkle chopped fresh basil, salt, and pepper to taste.

Greek Yogurt Parfait

Ingredients:

- Greek yogurt
- Fresh berries (blueberries, strawberries, raspberries)

- Honey

- Granola

- Almonds, sliced

Instructions:

1. Lay the Greek yogurt in either a glass or a bowl

2. Add a layer of fresh berries.

3. Drizzle with honey.

4. Sprinkle granola and sliced almonds on top.

Mediterranean Omelets

Ingredients:

- Eggs

- Spinach, chopped

- Feta cheese, crumbled

- Cherry tomatoes, halved

- Kalamata olives, sliced

- Olive oil

- Salt and pepper to taste

Instructions:

1. In a mixing dish, whisk together the eggs and season with salt and pepper..

2. Heat olive oil in a pan over medium heat.

3. Add chopped spinach and cook until wilted.

4. Pour the whisked eggs into the pan.

5. As the edges set, add feta cheese, cherry tomatoes, and olives.

6. Fold the omelet and cook until eggs are fully set.

Chia Seed Pudding

Ingredients:

- Chia seeds

- Almond milk

- Greek yogurt

- Honey

- Fresh fruit (figs, berries)

- Pistachios, chopped

Instructions:

1. Mix chia seeds with almond milk and let it sit in the fridge overnight.

2. In the morning, layer the chia pudding with Greek yogurt.

3. Drizzle with honey.

4. Top with fresh fruit and chopped pistachios.

Whole Grain Mediterranean Pancakes

Ingredients:

- Whole grain flour

- Milk (dairy or plant-based)

- Eggs

- Baking powder

- Orange zest

- Fresh fruit (oranges, berries)

- Greek yogurt

Instructions:

1. Mix whole grain flour, milk, eggs, baking powder, and orange zest to make the pancake batter.

2. Pancakes should be cooked on a griddle until golden brown..

3. Serve with fresh fruit along with Greek yogurt on the side.

Mediterranean Breakfast Wrap

Ingredients:

- Whole wheat tortilla

- Hummus

- Baby spinach

- Red bell pepper, sliced

- Cucumber, thinly sliced

- Cherry tomatoes, halved

- Feta cheese, crumbled

Instructions:

1. Spread hummus on the whole wheat tortilla.

2. Layer with baby spinach, red bell pepper, cucumber, cherry tomatoes, and feta cheese.

3. Roll into a wrap and enjoy.

Quinoa Breakfast Bowl

Ingredients:

- Cooked quinoa

- Almond milk

- Banana, sliced

- Pomegranate seeds

- Walnuts, chopped

- Cinnamon

Instructions:

1. Mix cooked quinoa with almond milk.

2. Top with banana slices, pomegranate seeds, and chopped walnuts.

3. Sprinkle with cinnamon for added flavor.

Mediterranean Frittata Cups

Ingredients:

- Eggs

- Spinach, chopped

- Cherry tomatoes, halved

- Red onion, finely chopped

- Feta cheese, crumbled

- Oregano

- Salt and pepper to taste

Instructions:

1. Preheat the oven and grease a muffin tin.

2. In a bowl, whisk eggs and add chopped spinach, cherry tomatoes, red onion, feta cheese, oregano, salt, and pepper.

3. Pour the mixture into muffin cups.

4. Bake until frittata cups are set and golden brown.

Smoothie Bowl

Ingredients:

- Frozen mixed berries

- Greek yogurt

- Banana

- Almond milk

- Chia seeds

- Granola

- Mint leaves for garnish

Instructions:

1. Blend frozen berries, Greek yogurt, banana, and almond milk until smooth.

2. Pour the smoothie into a bowl.

3. Top with chia seeds, granola, and garnish with mint leaves.

Open-Faced Caprese Breakfast Sandwich

Ingredients:

- Whole grain bread

- Tomato slices

- Fresh mozzarella

- Basil leaves

- Balsamic glaze

- Olive oil

- Salt and pepper to taste

Instructions:

1. Toast whole grain bread slices.

2. Layer with tomato slices, fresh mozzarella, and basil leaves.

3. Drizzle with balsamic glaze and olive oil.

4. Sprinkle with salt and pepper to taste.

Friendly Lunch Recipes

Grilled Chicken Greek Salad

Ingredients:

- Chicken breast, grilled and sliced
- Romaine lettuce, chopped
- Cucumber, sliced
- Cherry tomatoes, halved
- Kalamata olives, sliced
- Red onion, thinly sliced
- Feta cheese, crumbled
- Olive oil
- Lemon juice
- Oregano
- Salt and pepper to taste

Instructions:

1. In a large bowl, combine lettuce, cucumber, cherry tomatoes, olives, and red onion.
2. Top with grilled chicken and feta cheese.
3. Drizzle with olive oil and lemon juice.
4. Sprinkle with oregano, salt, and pepper. Toss gently to combine.

Mediterranean Quinoa Salad

Ingredients:

- Cooked quinoa

- Chickpeas, drained and rinsed

- Cucumber, diced

- Cherry tomatoes, quartered

- Red bell pepper, diced

- Red onion, finely chopped

- Feta cheese, crumbled

- Kalamata olives, sliced

- Olive oil

- Red wine vinegar

- Fresh parsley, chopped

- Salt and pepper to taste

Instructions:

1. In a large bowl, combine quinoa, chickpeas, cucumber, tomatoes, bell pepper, red onion, feta cheese, and olives.

2. In a small mixing bowl, combine the olive oil, red wine vinegar, parsley, salt, and pepper.

3. Combine the salad with the dressing to mix.

Mediterranean Stuffed Bell Peppers

Ingredients:

- Bell peppers, halved and cleaned
- Lean ground turkey
- Quinoa, cooked
- Cherry tomatoes, diced
- Spinach, chopped
- Feta cheese, crumbled
- Garlic, minced
- Olive oil
- Oregano
- Salt and pepper to taste

Instructions:

1. Preheat the oven and place halved bell peppers in a baking dish.
2. In a pan, cook ground turkey until browned. Add minced garlic, cherry tomatoes, and spinach.
3. Stir in cooked quinoa and feta cheese. Season with oregano, salt, and pepper.
4. Stuff each bell pepper half with the turkey and quinoa mixture.
5. Bake until peppers are tender.

Lentil Soup

Ingredients:

- Lentils, rinsed and drained
- Onion, chopped
- Carrots, diced
- Celery, diced
- Garlic, minced
- Tomatoes, diced
- Vegetable broth
- Olive oil
- Cumin
- Paprika
- Lemon juice
- Fresh parsley, chopped
- Salt and pepper to taste

Instructions:

1. In a large pot, sauté onion, carrots, celery, and garlic in olive oil until softened.

2. Add lentils, tomatoes, vegetable broth, cumin, paprika, salt, and pepper.

3. Simmer until lentils are tender.

Stir in lemon juice and garnish with fresh parsley before serving.

Tuna Salad Wrap

Ingredients:

- Canned tuna, drained
- Whole wheat wrap
- Greek yogurt
- Cucumber, sliced
- Cherry tomatoes, halved
- Red onion, thinly sliced
- Kalamata olives, sliced
- Spinach leaves
- Olive oil
- Lemon juice
- Oregano
- Salt and pepper to taste

Instructions:

1. In a bowl, mix tuna, Greek yogurt, cucumber, tomatoes, red onion, and olives.
2. Lay out a whole wheat wrap and place spinach leaves on it.
3. Spoon the tuna mixture onto the wrap.
4. Drizzle with olive oil and lemon juice. Sprinkle with oregano, salt, and pepper.
5. Roll the wrap and slice before serving.

Mediterranean Chicken Pita Pocket

Ingredients:

- Grilled chicken breast, sliced
- Whole wheat pita bread
- Hummus
- Tzatziki sauce
- Cherry tomatoes, halved
- Cucumber, sliced
- Red onion, thinly sliced
- Fresh mint leaves

Instructions:

1. Warm the pita bread.
2. Spread hummus and tzatziki sauce inside the pita.
3. Fill the pocket with grilled chicken, cherry tomatoes, cucumber, red onion, and fresh mint.

Vegetable and Quinoa Bowl

Ingredients:

- Cooked quinoa
- Eggplant, diced
- Zucchini, sliced
- Red bell pepper, diced
- Cherry tomatoes, halved
- Red onion, thinly sliced

- Feta cheese, crumbled
- Olive oil
- Balsamic vinegar
- Fresh basil, chopped
- Salt and pepper to taste

Instructions:

1. Roast eggplant, zucchini, red bell pepper, and red onion in olive oil until tender.
2. In a bowl, combine the cooked quinoa, roasted vegetables, cherry tomatoes, and feta cheese.
3. Drizzle with balsamic vinegar, sprinkle with fresh basil, salt, and pepper. Toss gently to combine.

Shrimp and Orzo Salad

Ingredients:

- Orzo pasta, cooked
- Shrimp, cooked and peeled
- Cherry tomatoes, halved
- Kalamata olives, sliced
- Feta cheese, crumbled
- Red onion, finely chopped
- Olive oil
- Lemon juice
- Oregano

- Salt and pepper to taste

Instructions:

1. In a large bowl, mix cooked orzo, shrimp, cherry tomatoes, olives, feta cheese, and red onion.

2. Drizzle with olive oil and lemon juice.

3. Sprinkle with oregano, salt, and pepper. Toss gently to combine.

Chickpea Salad

Ingredients:

- Chickpeas, drained and rinsed

- Cucumber, diced

- Cherry tomatoes, halved

- Red bell pepper, diced

- Red onion, finely chopped

- Feta cheese, crumbled

- Olive oil

- Red wine vinegar

- Fresh parsley, chopped

- Oregano

- Salt and pepper to taste

Instructions:

1. In a large bowl, combine chickpeas, cucumber, tomatoes, bell pepper, red onion, and feta cheese.

2. In a small bowl, whisk together olive oil, red wine vinegar, parsley, oregano, salt, and pepper.

3. Combine the salad with the dressing to mix.

Mediterranean Stuffed Portobello Mushrooms

Ingredients:

- Portobello mushrooms, stems removed
- Quinoa, cooked
- Spinach, sautéed
- Sun-dried tomatoes, chopped
- Feta cheese, crumbled
- Garlic, minced
- Olive oil
- Balsamic glaze
- Fresh basil, chopped
- Salt and pepper to taste

Instructions:

1. Preheat the oven and brush portobello mushrooms with olive oil.

2. In a bowl, mix cooked quinoa, sautéed spinach, sun-dried tomatoes, feta cheese, and minced garlic.

3. Stuff each mushroom with the quinoa mixture.

4. Bake until mushrooms are tender.

5. Drizzle with balsamic glaze and garnish with fresh basil before serving.

Enjoy these flavorful and nutritious Mediterranean-inspired lunch recipes as part of your weight loss journey!

Delicious Dinner Recipes

Mediterranean Baked Salmon

Ingredients:

- Salmon fillets
- Cherry tomatoes, halved
- Kalamata olives, sliced
- Red onion, thinly sliced
- Garlic, minced
- Olive oil
- Lemon juice
- Oregano
- Salt and pepper to taste

Instructions:

1. Preheat the oven to 400°F and arrange the salmon fillets on a baking sheet.

2. In a bowl, mix cherry tomatoes, olives, red onion, garlic, olive oil, lemon juice, oregano, salt, and pepper.

3. Spoon the tomato mixture over the salmon.

4. Bake until the salmon is cooked through.

Mediterranean Quinoa-Stuffed Bell Peppers

Ingredients:

- Bell peppers, halved and cleaned

- Quinoa, cooked

- Chickpeas, drained and rinsed

- Spinach, chopped

- Feta cheese, crumbled

- Tomatoes, diced

- Red onion, finely chopped

- Olive oil

- Lemon juice

- Oregano

- Salt and pepper to taste

Instructions:

1. Preheat the oven and place bell peppers in a baking dish.

2. In a bowl, mix quinoa, chickpeas, spinach, feta cheese, tomatoes, red onion, olive oil, lemon juice, oregano, salt, and pepper.

3. Stuff each bell pepper half with the quinoa mixture.

4. Bake until peppers are tender.

Mediterranean Grilled Chicken Skewers

Ingredients:

- Chicken breast, cut into chunks

- Zucchini, sliced

- Cherry tomatoes

- Red bell pepper, diced

- Red onion, cut into wedges

- Olive oil

- Lemon juice

- Garlic, minced

- Oregano

- Salt and pepper to taste

Instructions:

1. In a bowl, marinate chicken chunks, zucchini, cherry tomatoes, bell pepper, and red onion in olive oil, lemon juice, minced garlic, oregano, salt, and pepper.

2. Thread the marinated ingredients onto skewers.

3. Grill until the chicken is done and the vegetables are tender.

Lentil and Vegetable Stew

Ingredients:

- Brown lentils, rinsed and drained

- Carrots, diced

- Celery, diced

- Onion, chopped

- Garlic, minced

- Tomatoes, diced

- Vegetable broth

- Olive oil

- Cumin

- Paprika

- Fresh parsley, chopped

- Lemon wedges

- Salt and pepper to taste

Instructions:

1. In a pot, sauté onion, carrots, celery, and garlic in olive oil until softened.

2. Add lentils, tomatoes, vegetable broth, cumin, paprika, salt, and pepper.

3. Simmer until lentils are tender.

4. Serve with lemon wedges and garnished with fresh parsley.

Shrimp and Couscous

Ingredients:

- Shrimp, peeled and deveined
- Whole wheat couscous, cooked
- Cherry tomatoes, halved
- Cucumber, diced
- Red bell pepper, diced
- Red onion, finely chopped
- Feta cheese, crumbled
- Olive oil
- Lemon juice
- Fresh mint leaves, chopped
- Salt and pepper to taste

Instructions:

1. In a pan, sauté shrimp in olive oil until cooked.
2. In a bowl, mix cooked couscous, cherry tomatoes, cucumber, bell pepper, red onion, feta cheese, olive oil, lemon juice, mint leaves, salt, and pepper.
3. Top the couscous mixture with sautéed shrimp before serving.

Eggplant and Chickpea Stew

Ingredients:

- Eggplant, diced

- Chickpeas, drained and rinsed

- Tomatoes, diced

- Red onion, finely chopped

- Garlic, minced

- Olive oil

- Vegetable broth

- Cumin

- Paprika

- Fresh parsley, chopped

- Lemon wedges

- Salt and pepper to taste

Instructions:

1. In a pot, sauté eggplant, chickpeas, tomatoes, red onion, and garlic in olive oil until softened.

2. Add vegetable broth, cumin, paprika, salt, and pepper. Simmer until eggplant is tender.

3. Serve with lemon wedges and garnished with fresh parsley.

Turkey and Vegetable Stir-Fry

Ingredients:

- Ground turkey

- Broccoli florets

- Red bell pepper, sliced

- Cherry tomatoes, halved

- Zucchini, sliced

- Garlic, minced

- Olive oil

- Lemon juice

- Oregano

- Fresh basil, chopped

- Salt and pepper to taste

Instructions:

1. In a pan, cook ground turkey in olive oil until browned.

2. Add broccoli, bell pepper, tomatoes, zucchini, minced garlic, lemon juice, oregano, salt, and pepper.

3. Stir-fry until vegetables are tender.

4. Garnish with fresh basil before serving.

Baked Cod with Tomatoes and Olives

Ingredients:

- Cod fillets

- Cherry tomatoes, halved

- Kalamata olives, sliced

- Red onion, thinly sliced

- Olive oil

- Lemon juice

- Garlic, minced

- Oregano

- Salt and pepper to taste

Instructions:

1. Preheat the oven and place cod fillets on a baking sheet.

2. In a bowl, mix cherry tomatoes, olives, red onion, olive oil, lemon juice, minced garlic, oregano, salt, and pepper.

3. Spoon the tomato mixture over the cod.

4. Bake until the cod is cooked through.

Chickpea and Spinach Stuffed Sweet Potatoes

Ingredients:

- Sweet potatoes, baked

- Chickpeas, drained and rinsed

- Spinach, sautéed

- Feta cheese, crumbled

- Olive oil

- Lemon juice

- Garlic, minced

- Oregano

- Salt and pepper to taste

Instructions:

1. Cut open baked sweet potatoes and fluff the insides with a fork.

2. In a bowl, mix chickpeas, sautéed spinach, feta cheese, olive oil, lemon juice, minced garlic, oregano, salt, and pepper.

3. Stuff the sweet potatoes with the chickpea mixture.

Stuffed Zucchini Boats

Ingredients:

- Zucchini, halved lengthwise

- Ground turkey

- Quinoa, cooked

- Cherry tomatoes, diced

- Feta cheese, crumbled

- Olive oil

- Lemon juice

- Oregano

- Salt and pepper to taste

Instructions:

1. Preheat the oven and scoop out the insides of zucchini halves.

2. In a pan, cook ground turkey in olive oil until browned.

3. Mix cooked quinoa, diced tomatoes, feta cheese, olive oil, lemon juice, oregano, salt, and pepper with the turkey.

4. Stuff the zucchini halves with the mixture and bake until zucchini is tender.

Healthy Snack Recipes

Hummus with Veggie Sticks

Ingredients:

- Hummus (store-bought or homemade)
- Carrot sticks
- Cucumber slices
- Cherry tomatoes

Instructions:

1. Arrange carrot sticks, cucumber slices, and cherry tomatoes on a plate.
2. Serve with a side of hummus for dipping.

Greek Yogurt and Berry Parfait

Ingredients:

- Greek yogurt
- Mixed berries (blueberries, strawberries, raspberries)
- Honey
- Almonds, sliced

Instructions:

1. Lay the Greek yogurt in either a glass or a bowl
2. Add a layer of mixed berries.
3. Drizzle with honey and sprinkle sliced almonds on top.

Guacamole with Whole Wheat Pita

Ingredients:

- Avocado, mashed

- Tomato, diced

- Red onion, finely chopped

- Garlic, minced

- Cilantro, chopped

- Lime juice

- Whole wheat pita, cut into wedges

Instructions:

1. In a bowl, mix mashed avocado, tomato, red onion, garlic, cilantro, and lime juice.

2. Serve with whole wheat pita wedges.

Mediterranean Trail Mix

Ingredients:

- Almonds

- Walnuts

- Pistachios

- Dried apricots, chopped

- Dark chocolate chips

Instructions:

1. Combine almonds, walnuts, pistachios, dried apricots, and dark chocolate chips in a bowl.

2. Mix well and portion into snack-sized servings.

Stuffed Grape Leaves (Dolma) with Greek Yogurt Sauce

Ingredients:

- Grape leaves (canned or fresh)

- Quinoa, cooked

- Chickpeas, drained and rinsed

- Tomatoes, diced

- Red onion, finely chopped

- Feta cheese, crumbled

- Greek yogurt

- Lemon juice

- Dill, chopped

Instructions:

1. Lay out grape leaves and fill each with a mixture of cooked quinoa, chickpeas, tomatoes, red onion, and feta cheese.

2. Roll the grapes leaves and serve with a dipping sauce made from Greek yogurt, lemon juice, and chopped dill.

Mediterranean Caprese Skewers

Ingredients:

- Cherry tomatoes
- Fresh mozzarella balls
- Basil leaves
- Balsamic glaze

Instructions:

1. On small skewers, thread cherry tomatoes, fresh mozzarella balls, and ba sil leaves.

2. Drizzle with balsamic glaze before serving.

Mediterranean Cucumber Cups

Ingredients:

- Mini cucumbers
- Greek yogurt
- Kalamata olives, sliced
- Cherry tomatoes, diced
- Fresh mint, chopped

Instructions:

1. Cut mini cucumbers into small cups.

2. Fill each cup with a mixture of Greek yogurt, sliced Kalamata olives, diced cherry tomatoes, and chopped fresh mint.

Mediterranean Roasted Chickpeas

Ingredients:

- Chickpeas, drained and rinsed
- Olive oil
- Smoked paprika
- Garlic powder
- Cumin
- Salt and pepper to taste

Instructions:

1. Preheat the oven and toss chickpeas with olive oil, smoked paprika, garlic powder, cumin, salt, and pepper.
2. Roast until chickpeas are crispy.

Cottage Cheese Bowl

Ingredients:

- Cottage cheese
- Pineapple chunks
- Almonds, sliced
- Mint leaves, chopped

Instructions:

1. In a bowl, combine cottage cheese, pineapple chunks, sliced almonds, and chopped mint.
2. Mix well and enjoy.

Dill Yogurt Dip with Pita Chips

Ingredients:

- Greek yogurt

- Fresh dill, chopped

- Lemon juice

- Garlic, minced

- Olive oil

- Whole wheat pita, cut into triangles

Instructions:

1. In a bowl, mix Greek yogurt, chopped dill, lemon juice, minced garlic, and a drizzle of olive oil.

2. Serve the dip with whole wheat pita chips.

Nutritious Dessert Recipes

Mediterranean Fresh Fruit Salad

Ingredients:

- Mixed fruits (such as berries, melons, and citrus)
- Mint leaves, chopped
- Honey

Instructions:

1. Chop the mixed fruits and combine them in a bowl.
2. Sprinkle with chopped mint leaves.
3. Drizzle with honey and toss gently to coat.

Greek Yogurt and Berry Popsicles

Ingredients:

- Greek yogurt
- Mixed berries (blueberries, strawberries, raspberries)
- Honey

Instructions:

1. Combine Greek yogurt and honey in a mixing basin.
2. Layer the yogurt mixture and mixed berries in popsicle molds.
3. Freeze until solid.

Orange and Olive Oil Cake

Ingredients:

- Oranges, juiced and zested
- Olive oil
- Eggs
- Almond flour
- Baking powder
- Honey

Instructions:

1. Preheat the oven to 350°F and lightly butter a cake pan.
2. In a bowl, mix orange juice, orange zest, olive oil, eggs, almond flour, baking powder, and honey.
3. Pour the batter into the cake pan and bake until a toothpick comes out clean.

Yogurt Parfait with Pistachios

Ingredients:

- Greek yogurt
- Pistachios, chopped
- Dried figs, chopped
- Honey

Instructions:

1. Lay the Greek yogurt in either a glass or a bowl

2. Add chopped pistachios and dried figs.

3. Drizzle with honey.

Chia Seed Pudding with Almond Milk

Ingredients:

- Chia seeds

- Almond milk

- Pomegranate seeds

- Pistachios, chopped

Instructions:

1. Mix chia seeds with almond milk and let it sit in the fridge until it thickens.

2. Layer the chia pudding with pomegranate seeds and chopped pistachios.

Honey and Walnut Baklava

Ingredients:

- Phyllo dough

- Walnuts, chopped

- Honey

- Cinnamon

- Olive oil

Instructions:

1. Preheat the oven and layer phyllo dough in a baking dish, brushing each layer with olive oil.

2. Mix chopped walnuts with cinnamon and spread over the phyllo layers.

3. Continue layering until all ingredients are used.

4. After baking till golden brown, drizzle with honey.

Grilled Peaches with Yogurt

Ingredients:

- Peaches, halved and pitted

- Greek yogurt

- Honey

- Mint leaves, chopped

Instructions:

1. Preheat the grill and grill peach halves until they have grill marks.

2. Serve each grilled peach with a dollop of Greek yogurt.

3. Drizzle with honey and top with mint leaves.

Dark Chocolate-Dipped Strawberries

Ingredients:

- Strawberries

- Dark chocolate, melted

- Almonds, chopped

Instructions:

1. Dip each strawberry into melted dark chocolate.

2. Place on a parchment-lined tray and sprinkle with chopped almonds.

3. Allow the chocolate to set before serving.

Almond and Orange Biscotti

Ingredients:

- Almonds, chopped

- Almond flour

- Orange zest

- Honey

- Eggs

- Baking powder

Instructions:

1. Preheat the oven and mix chopped almonds, almond flour, orange zest, honey, eggs, and baking powder in a bowl.

2. Shape the dough into a log and bake until golden brown.

3. Slice into biscotti shapes.

Mediterranean Lemon Sorbet

Ingredients:

- Lemons, juiced and zested

- Water

- Honey

- Mint leaves, for garnish

Instructions:

1. In a saucepan, heat water and honey until the honey dissolves.

2. Let the mixture cool, and then add lemon juice and zest.

3. Pour into an ice cream machine and freeze until solid

4. Garnish with mint leaves before serving

Fruits and Smoothie Recipes

Green Goddess Smoothie

Ingredients:

- Spinach
- Cucumber, peeled and sliced
- Greek yogurt
- Green apple, cored and chopped
- Mint leaves
- Ice cubes

Instructions:

1. Blend spinach, cucumber, Greek yogurt, green apple, mint leaves, and ice cubes until smooth.

Citrus and Berry Mediterranean Smoothie

Ingredients:

- Oranges, peeled and segmented
- Mixed berries (blueberries, strawberries, raspberries)
- Greek yogurt
- Almond milk
- Chia seeds

Instructions:

1. Blend oranges, mixed berries, Greek yogurt, almond milk, and chia seeds until well combined.

Mango and Pineapple Smoothie

Ingredients:

- Mango, peeled and diced

- Pineapple, diced

- Greek yogurt

- Coconut water

- Flaxseeds

Instructions:

1. Blend mango, pineapple, Greek yogurt, coconut water, and flaxseeds until smooth.

Avocado and Banana Smoothie

Ingredients:

- Avocado, peeled and pitted

- Banana

- Spinach

- Greek yogurt

- Almond milk

- Honey

Instructions:

1. Blend avocado, banana, spinach, Greek yogurt, almond milk, and honey until creamy.

Greek Yogurt and Berry Protein Smoothie

Ingredients:

- Greek yogurt

- Mixed berries (blueberries, strawberries, raspberries)

- Protein powder

- Almond milk

- Walnuts, chopped

Instructions:

1. Blend Greek yogurt, mixed berries, protein powder, almond milk, and chopped walnuts until well mixed.

Pineapple and Kale Smoothie

Ingredients:

- Pineapple, diced

- Kale leaves, stems removed

- Greek yogurt

- Coconut water

- Chia seeds

Instructions:

1. Blend pineapple, kale, Greek yogurt, coconut water, and chia seeds until smooth.

Berry and Almond Butter Smoothie

Ingredients:

- Mixed berries (blueberries, strawberries, raspberries)

- Almond butter

- Greek yogurt

- Almond milk

- Flaxseeds

Instructions:

1. Blend mixed berries, almond butter, Greek yogurt, almond milk, and flaxseeds until creamy.

Peach and Mint Smoothie

Ingredients:

- Peaches, peeled and sliced

- Mint leaves

- Greek yogurt

- Coconut water

- Ice cubes

Instructions:

1. Blend peaches, mint leaves, Greek yogurt, coconut water, and ice cubes until well combined.

Watermelon and Cucumber Smoothie

Ingredients:

- Watermelon, diced

- Cucumber, peeled and sliced

- Greek yogurt

- Lime juice

- Basil leaves

Instructions:

1. Blend watermelon, cucumber, Greek yogurt, lime juice, and basil leaves until smooth.

Chocolate Banana Protein Smoothie

Ingredients:

- Banana

- Greek yogurt

- Cocoa powder

- Almond milk

- Protein powder

Instructions:

1. Blend banana, Greek yogurt, cocoa powder, almond milk, and protein powder until well mixed.

Healthy Vegetarian Recipes

Quinoa Salad with Chickpeas

Ingredients:

- Quinoa, cooked
- Chickpeas, drained and rinsed
- Cherry tomatoes, halved
- Cucumber, diced
- Red bell pepper, diced
- Red onion, finely chopped
- Feta cheese, crumbled
- Kalamata olives, sliced
- Olive oil
- Lemon juice
- Oregano
- Salt and pepper to taste

Instructions:

1. In a large bowl, combine cooked quinoa, chickpeas, tomatoes, cucumber, bell pepper, red onion, feta cheese, and olives.

2. In a small bowl, whisk together olive oil, lemon juice, oregano, salt, and pepper.

3. Combine the salad with the dressing to mix.

Eggplant and Tomato Bake

Ingredients:

- Eggplant, sliced
- Tomatoes, sliced
- Garlic, minced
- Olive oil
- Basil leaves, chopped
- Feta cheese, crumbled
- Oregano
- Salt and pepper to taste

Instructions:

1. Preheat the oven and layer sliced eggplant and tomatoes in a baking dish.

2. Drizzle with olive oil, sprinkle minced garlic, basil leaves, feta cheese, oregano, salt, and pepper.

3. Bake until the vegetables are tender.

Lentil and Vegetable Stew

Ingredients:

- Brown lentils, rinsed and drained
- Carrots, diced
- Celery, diced
- Onion, chopped
- Garlic, minced

- Tomatoes, diced
- Vegetable broth
- Olive oil
- Cumin
- Paprika
- Fresh parsley, chopped
- Lemon wedges
- Salt and pepper to taste

Instructions:

1. In a large pot, sauté onion, carrots, celery, and garlic in olive oil until softened.

2. Add lentils, tomatoes, vegetable broth, cumin, paprika, salt, and pepper.

3. Simmer until lentils are tender.

4. Stir in lemon juice and garnish with fresh parsley before serving.

Chickpea and Spinach Stuffed Sweet Potatoes

Ingredients:

- Sweet potatoes, baked
- Chickpeas, drained and rinsed
- Spinach, sautéed
- Feta cheese, crumbled
- Olive oil
- Lemon juice

- Garlic, minced

- Oregano

- Salt and pepper to taste

Instructions:

1. Cut open baked sweet potatoes and fluff the insides with a fork.

2. In a bowl, mix chickpeas, sautéed spinach, feta cheese, olive oil, lemon juice, minced garlic, oregano, salt, and pepper.

3. Stuff the sweet potatoes with the chickpea mixture.

Caprese Zucchini Noodles

Ingredients:

- Zucchini, spiralized into noodles

- Cherry tomatoes, halved

- Fresh mozzarella balls

- Basil leaves, torn

- Olive oil

- Balsamic glaze

- Salt and pepper to taste

Instructions:

1. In a pan, sauté zucchini noodles until just tender.

2. Toss with cherry tomatoes, fresh mozzarella balls, torn basil leaves, olive oil, balsamic glaze, salt, and pepper.

Greek Salad Wrap

Ingredients:

- Whole wheat wrap
- Romaine lettuce, chopped
- Cherry tomatoes, halved
- Cucumber, sliced
- Red onion, thinly sliced
- Feta cheese, crumbled
- Kalamata olives, sliced
- Greek dressing

Instructions:

1. Lay out a whole wheat wrap and place lettuce, tomatoes, cucumber, red onion, feta cheese, and olives on it.
2. Drizzle with Greek dressing.
3. Roll the wrap and slice before serving.

Stuffed Bell Peppers with Quinoa

Ingredients:

- Bell peppers, halved and cleaned
- Quinoa, cooked
- Cherry tomatoes, diced
- Kalamata olives, sliced
- Red onion, finely chopped
- Feta cheese, crumbled

- Olive oil

- Lemon juice

- Oregano

- Salt and pepper to taste

Instructions:

1. Preheat the oven and place bell peppers in a baking dish.

2. In a bowl, mix cooked quinoa, tomatoes, olives, red onion, feta cheese, olive oil, lemon juice, oregano, salt, and pepper.

3. Stuff each bell pepper half with the quinoa mixture.

4. Bake until peppers are tender.

Spinach and Feta Stuffed Mushrooms

Ingredients:

- Mushrooms, stems removed

- Spinach, sautéed

- Feta cheese, crumbled

- Garlic, minced

- Olive oil

- Lemon juice

- Oregano

- Salt and pepper to taste

Instructions:

1. Preheat the oven and brush mushroom caps with olive oil.

2. In a bowl, mix sautéed spinach, feta cheese, minced garlic, olive oil, lemon juice, oregano, salt, and pepper.

3. Stuff each mushroom with the mixture and bake until mushrooms are tender.

Mediterranean Chickpea Salad

Ingredients:

- Chickpeas, drained and rinsed
- Cucumber, diced
- Cherry tomatoes, halved
- Red bell pepper, diced
- Red onion, finely chopped
- Feta cheese, crumbled
- Olive oil
- Red wine vinegar
- Fresh parsley, chopped
- Oregano
- Salt and pepper to taste

Instructions:

1. In a large bowl, combine chickpeas, cucumber, tomatoes, bell pepper, red onion, and feta cheese.

2. In a small bowl, whisk together olive oil, red wine vinegar, parsley, oregano, salt, and pepper.

3. Combine the salad with the dressing to mix.

Lentil and Vegetable Skewers

Ingredients:

- Cooked lentils

- Zucchini, sliced

- Cherry tomatoes

- Red onion, cut into wedges

- Bell peppers, diced

- Olive oil

- Lemon juice

- Garlic, minced

- Oregano

- Salt and pepper to taste

Instructions:

1. In a bowl, marinate cooked lentils, zucchini, cherry tomatoes, red onion, and bell peppers in olive oil, lemon juice, minced garlic, oregano, salt, and pepper.

2. Thread the marinated ingredients onto skewers.

3. Grill until the vegetables are tender.

Tips for Dining Out While On the Diet

1. Choose Mediterranean Restaurants:

Opt for restaurants that offer Mediterranean cuisine or have a variety of fresh, whole foods on their menu.

2. Start with a Salad:

Begin your meal with a salad loaded with a variety of colorful vegetables. Ask for olive oil and vinegar on the side for dressing.

3. Prioritize Seafood:

Select fish or seafood dishes, preferably grilled or baked. These alternatives are high in omega-3 fatty acids.

4. Select Lean Proteins:

Choose lean protein sources such as grilled chicken, turkey, or legumes. Avoid fried and heavily processed meats.

5. Include Whole Grains:

Opt for dishes that incorporate whole grains, such as whole wheat pasta, quinoa, or brown rice.

6. Customize Your Order:

Don't hesitate to customize your order. Ask for adjustments like substituting sides for more vegetables or choosing whole grain options.

7. Watch Portion Sizes:

Be mindful of portion sizes, and consider sharing dishes with dining companions. You can also ask for a to-go box upfront and save a portion for later.

8. Limit Bread and Choose Whole Grain:

If bread is served before the meal, limit your intake. If available, choose whole-grain options.

9. Embrace Vegetable-Based Dishes:

Explore vegetarian or vegetable-based dishes, such as ratatouille, stuffed peppers, or eggplant dishes.

Integrating Exercise into a Mediterranean lifestyle

1. Outdoor Activities:

- Take advantage of the Mediterranean climate by engaging in outdoor activities. Walks along the beach, hiking, cycling, or jogging in scenic areas can be both enjoyable and physically beneficial.

2. Active Commuting:

- Consider incorporating active modes of transportation into your daily routine. Walk or bike to work, or use public transportation that involves some walking.

3. Social Exercise:

- Engage in physical activities with friends and family. Play sports together, join a local sports club, or participate in group fitness classes.

4. Embrace Traditional Activities:

- Participate in traditional Mediterranean activities that involve physical exertion, such as dancing or gardening.

5. Incorporate Regular Walks:

- Make walking a daily habit. Take post-meal strolls, explore your neighborhood, and use walking as a means of relaxation and stress reduction.

6. Yoga and Mindful Movement:

- Practice yoga or other mindful movement exercises. These alternatives are high in omega-3 fatty acids.

7. Swimming:

- Take advantage of the Mediterranean Sea or local pools for swimming.

8. Interval Training:

- Incorporate high-intensity interval training (HIIT) into your routine. Short bursts of intense exercise followed by periods of rest can be time-efficient and effective for fitness.

9. Dance Classes:

- Join dance classes or dance socially. Traditional Mediterranean dances or more contemporary styles can be a fun way to stay active.

Types of Exercise that Complement the diet for Weight Loss

1. Cardiovascular Exercise:

- **Benefits:**

  - Burns calories.

  - Improves cardiovascular health.

- **Examples:**

  - Walking or brisk walking.

  - Running or jogging.

  - Cycling.

  - Swimming.

  - Dancing.

2. High-Intensity Interval Training (HIIT):

- **Benefits:**

  - Efficient calorie burning.

  - Boosts metabolism.

- **Examples:**

  - Short bursts of intense exercises (e.g., sprinting, jumping jacks) followed by rest periods.

3. Strength Training:

- **Benefits:**

  - Builds lean muscle mass, which increases metabolism.

  - Enhances overall strength and endurance.

- **Examples:**

  - Weightlifting.

  - Bodyweight exercises (e.g., squats, lunges, push-ups).

  - Resistance band exercises.

4. Yoga:

- **Benefits:**

  - Improves flexibility and balance.

  - Reduces stress.

- **Examples:**

  - Hatha yoga.

  - Vinyasa yoga.

  - Power yoga.

5. Pilates:

- **Benefits:**
  - Strengthens core muscles.
  - Improves flexibility.
- **Examples:**
  - Mat Pilates.
  - Reformer Pilates.

6. Functional Training:

- **Benefits:**
  - Mimics real-life movements.
  - Improves overall functionality and coordination.
- **Examples:**
  - Functional fitness classes.
  - Exercises that involve multiple muscle groups (e.g., kettlebell swings, medicine ball slams).

7. Circuit Training:

- **Benefits:**
  - Combines strength and cardio.
  - Time-efficient.

- **Examples:**

  - Design a circuit with various exercises (e.g., jumping jacks, squats, push-ups) and perform each for a set amount of time before moving to the next.

8. Group Fitness Classes:

- **Benefits:**

  - Adds a social component to exercise.

  - Provides structure and guidance.

- **Examples:**

  - Group cycling classes.

  - Dance fitness classes.

  - Bootcamp classes.

9. Mind-Body Exercises:

- **Benefits:**

  - Promotes mindfulness and stress reduction.

- **Examples:**

  - Tai Chi.

  - Qigong.

10. Outdoor Activities:

- **Benefits:**

  - Adds variety to your routine.

- Increases enjoyment and motivation.

- **Examples:**

  - Hiking.

  - Trail running.

  - Kayaking.

11. Interval Walking:

- **Benefits:**

  - Effective for beginners.

  - It is simple to incorporate into regular habits.

- **Examples:**

  - Alternate between brisk walking and slower-paced walking.

12. Water Aerobics:

- **Benefits:**

  - Low-impact exercise.

  - Supports joint health.

- **Examples:**

  - Water aerobics classes.

  - Swimming laps.

13. Cycling:

- **Benefits:**

  - Low-impact on joints.

- Suitable for all fitness levels.

- **Examples:**

  - Cycling outdoors.

  - Indoor cycling classes.

14. Rowing:

- **Benefits:**

  - Full-body workout.

  - Cardiovascular and strength benefits.

- **Examples:**

  - Rowing machine workouts.

15. Dance Workouts:

- **Benefits:**

  - Fun and enjoyable.

  - Effective for burning calories.

- **Examples:**

  - Zumba.

  - Dance cardio workouts.

Benefits of Physical Activity beyond Weight Management

1. Cardiovascular Health:

- **Reduces Risk of Heart Disease:** Regular exercise helps maintain healthy blood pressure, cholesterol levels, and improves overall cardiovascular function, reducing the risk of heart disease.

2. Muscle and Bone Health:

- **Strengthens Muscles and Bones:** Weight-bearing exercises and resistance training enhance muscle strength and bone density, reducing the risk of osteoporosis and frailty.

3. Metabolic Health:

- **Improves Insulin Sensitivity:** Physical activity helps regulate blood sugar levels, improving insulin sensitivity and reducing the risk of type 2 diabetes.

4. Mental Health and Mood:

- **Reduces Stress and Anxiety:** Exercise triggers the release of endorphins, which are natural mood lifters, reducing stress and anxiety.

- **Improves Sleep:** Regular physical activity can enhance sleep quality and promote better sleep patterns.

5. Cognitive Function:

- **Enhances Brain Health:** Exercise is associated with improved cognitive function, memory, and a reduced risk of age-related cognitive decline.

6. Weight Management:

- **Promotes Healthy Weight:** While not the sole factor, exercise plays a crucial role in weight management by burning calories and supporting a healthy metabolism.

7. Joint Health:

- **Supports Joint Function:** Regular movement and exercise help maintain joint flexibility, reducing the risk of joint pain and stiffness.

8. Improved Immune Function:

- **Enhances Immune System:** Moderate, regular exercise has been linked to improved immune function, reducing the risk of illness.

9. Better Respiratory Function:

- **Strengthens Respiratory Muscles:** Exercise improves lung capacity and respiratory function, promoting better oxygen intake.

Overcoming Common Challenges

1. Lack of Time:

- **Strategy:** Prioritize and schedule activities. Divide your workouts into shorter periods throughout the day.

- Plan and prepare Mediterranean meals in batches for quick and convenient access.

2. Unrealistic Goals:

- **Strategy:** Set small, achievable goals. Focus on gradual rather than abrupt changes.

- Celebrate small victories and adjust goals as needed.

3. Social Pressure:

- **Strategy:** Communicate your goals with friends and family, so they can provide support. Educate others about the Mediterranean lifestyle, and find activities that align with your health goals when socializing.

4. Lack of Motivation:

- **Strategy:** Find activities you enjoy. Switch up your workout program to keep it fresh.

- Remind yourself of the health benefits and how good you feel after making healthy choices.

5. Busy Lifestyle:

- **Strategy:** Plan and prep meals in advance. Incorporate short, high-intensity workouts. Look for opportunities to move during the day, such as taking the stairs or walking during breaks.

6. Food Temptations:

- **Strategy:** Keep a variety of Mediterranean snacks on hand. Allow yourself occasional treats in moderation. Focus on the delicious and satisfying aspects of Mediterranean cuisine.

7. Limited Resources:

- **Strategy:** Use bodyweight exercises if you can't access a gym. Explore local markets for affordable Mediterranean ingredients. Utilize online resources for workout ideas and recipes.

8. Lack of Support:

- **Strategy:** Connect with like-minded individuals online or in local communities. Join fitness classes or groups. Share your journey with friends or family to build a support system.

9. Plateau in Progress:

- **Strategy:** Reevaluate your routine. Make adjustments to your workout intensity or try new activities. Experiment with different Mediterranean recipes to keep your meals exciting.

BONUS

30 Days Healthy Meal Plan

Day	Breakfast	Lunch	Dinner	Snack
1	Greek Yogurt Parfait	Mediterranean Quinoa Salad	Baked Cod with Tomatoes and Olives	Mixed Nuts
2	Oatmeal with Berries	Lentil and Vegetable Stew	Chickpea and Spinach Stuffed Sweet Potatoes	Hummus with Veggie Sticks
3	Mediterranean Frittata	Greek Salad Wrap	Grilled Chicken Skewers	Greek Yogurt and Berry Parfait
4	Smoothie (Spinach, Banana, Almond Milk)	Caprese Zucchini Noodles	Eggplant and Chickpea Stew	Greek Salad
5	Whole Wheat Toast with Avocado	Mediterranean Chickpea Salad	Lentil and Vegetable Skewers	Dark Chocolate-Dipped Strawberries
6	Scrambled Eggs with	Greek Lentil Soup	Mediterranean Quinoa-Stuffed	Greek Yogurt with Honey

Day	Breakfast	Lunch	Dinner	Snack
	Spinach		Bell Peppers	
7	Chia Seed Pudding with Berries	Mediterranean Chickpea and Spinach Stuffed Mushrooms	Grilled Peaches with Yogurt	Almonds
8	Greek Yogurt Smoothie with Mixed Berries	Mediterranean Chickpea and Spinach Stuffed Mushrooms	Mediterranean Stuffed Zucchini Boats	Greek Yogurt and Berry Popsicles
9	Mediterranean Omelets	Greek Lentil Salad	Mediterranean Baked Salmon	Fresh Fruit Salad
10	Whole Grain Pancakes with Maple Syrup	Mediterranean Quinoa Salad	Eggplant and Tomato Bake	Greek Yogurt with Almonds
11	Overnight Oats with Chia Seeds	Mediterranean Hummus Wrap	Mediterranean Chickpea Salad	Mixed Berries
12	Smoothie (Mango, Pineapple, Greek Yogurt)	Caprese Salad	Greek Stuffed Bell Peppers	Greek Yogurt and Walnut Baklava
13	Avocado Toast with Tomatoes	Mediterranean Stuffed Mushrooms	Mediterranean Baked Cod with Tomatoes and Olives	Mediterranean Trail Mix

Day	Breakfast	Lunch	Dinner	Snack
14	Mediterranean Frittata	Greek Salad Wrap	Lentil and Vegetable Stew	Greek Yogurt Parfait
15	Whole Wheat Toast with Hummus	Mediterranean Quinoa-Stuffed Bell Peppers	Grilled Chicken Skewers	Mediterranean Guacamole with Pita
16	Greek Yogurt Smoothie with Mixed Berries	Mediterranean Chickpea Salad	Mediterranean Lentil and Vegetable Skewers	Dark Chocolate-Dipped Strawberries
17	Oatmeal with Berries	Greek Lentil Soup	Eggplant and Chickpea Stew	Almonds
18	Scrambled Eggs with Spinach	Caprese Zucchini Noodles	Mediterranean Quinoa Salad	Greek Yogurt and Berry Parfait
19	Chia Seed Pudding with Berries	Greek Salad	Mediterranean Stuffed Zucchini Boats	Greek Yogurt with Honey
20	Greek Yogurt Parfait	Mediterranean Quinoa Salad	Baked Cod with Tomatoes and Olives	Mixed Nuts
21	Smoothie (Spinach, Banana, Almond Milk)	Chickpea and Spinach Stuffed Sweet Potatoes	Grilled Chicken Skewers	Hummus with Veggie Sticks

Day	Breakfast	Lunch	Dinner	Snack
22	Mediterranean Frittata	Lentil and Vegetable Stew	Chickpea and Spinach Stuffed Mushrooms	Greek Yogurt and Berry Popsicles
23	Whole Wheat Pancakes with Berries	Mediterranean Chickpea Salad	Mediterranean Lentil and Vegetable Skewers	Greek Yogurt with Almonds
24	Overnight Oats with Chia Seeds	Greek Salad Wrap	Mediterranean Baked Salmon	Fresh Fruit Salad
25	Avocado Toast with Tomatoes	Mediterranean Chickpea Salad	Grilled Peaches with Yogurt	Dark Chocolate-Dipped Strawberries
26	Smoothie (Mango, Pineapple, Greek Yogurt)	Caprese Salad	Greek Stuffed Bell Peppers	Greek Yogurt and Walnut Baklava
27	Mediterranean Omelets	Greek Lentil Salad	Mediterranean Quinoa-Stuffed Bell Peppers	Greek Yogurt Parfait
28	Whole Wheat Toast with Hummus	Mediterranean Stuffed Mushrooms	Mediterranean Baked Cod with Tomatoes and Olives	Mediterranean Trail Mix

Day	Breakfast	Lunch	Dinner	Snack
29	Greek Yogurt Smoothie with Mixed Berries	Mediterranean Chickpea and Spinach Stuffed Mushrooms	Eggplant and Tomato Bake	Almonds
30	Oatmeal with Berries	Greek Salad Wrap	Mediterranean Stuffed Zucchini Boats	Greek Yogurt with Honey

Feel free to adjust the ingredients and meals based on your preferences and dietary needs. Additionally, ensure to stay hydrated throughout the day by drinking plenty of water.